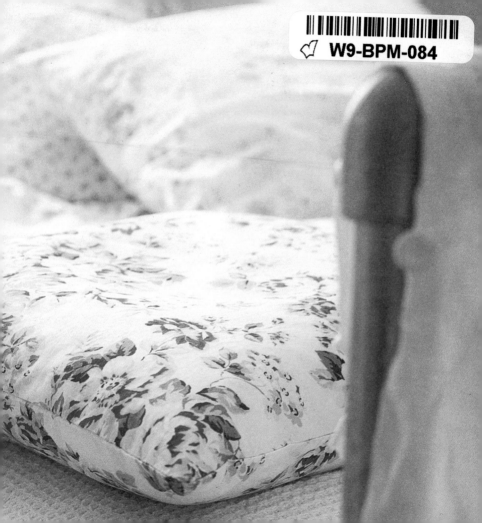

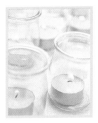

de-stress

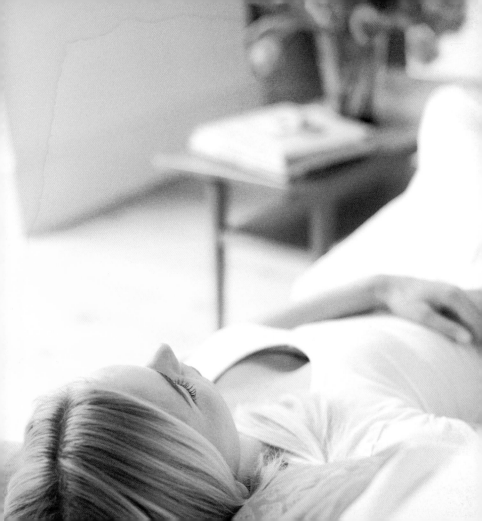

home spa

de-stress

Liz Wilde

RYLAND
PETERS
& SMALL
LONDON NEW YORK

Designer Sarah Fraser
Senior Editor Clare Double
Picture Researcher Tracy Ogino
Production Susannah Straughan
Art Director Gabriella Le Grazie
Publishing Director Alison Starling

First published in the United States
in 2005 by Ryland Peters & Small
519 Broadway
5th Floor
New York NY 10012
www.rylandpeters.com

Printed and bound in China

ISBN 1 84172 853 5

If you are in any doubt about your health, consult
your doctor before making any changes to your
usual dietary and wellbeing regime. Essential oils
are very powerful and potentially toxic if used too
liberally. Please follow the guidelines and never use
the oils neat on bare skin, unless advised otherwise.
This book is not suitable for anyone during pregnancy.

contents

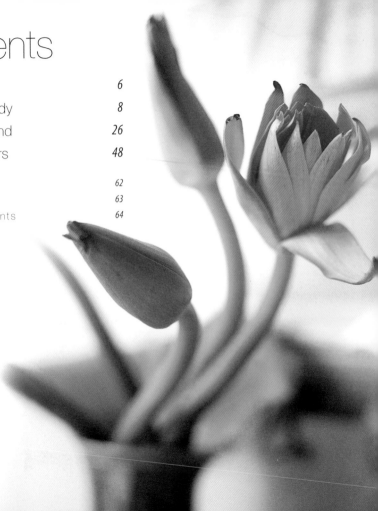

introduction

You'd be forgiven for thinking stress is unavoidable. A third of sick leave is blamed on stress, yet there's a big difference between people's ideas of what counts as stressful—which is why one person may find traveling by plane way too stressful, yet another takes up hang-gliding as a hobby! Stress really means any form of *distress* and has more to do

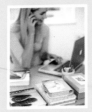 with your reaction to a situation than the situation itself. Stress affects both your mind and body. Remember the last time you ran for a bus. Your breathing quickened, your muscles tensed, and you may even have broken into a sweat. This is your body responding to an emergency, and exactly the same can happen when you're emotionally stressed. This "fight or flight" response once came in handy for attacking wild animals, but now does little more than put a strain on your body's defenses.

A little stress can be a good thing (you're more likely to pass an exam if you're anxious about doing well), but it's the stressful situations that last for weeks and months that can do you harm. Modern life is spent speeding up, so it makes sense that to reduce stress you need to learn techniques that slow you down. But to reduce stress long-term, you also need to change how you respond to situations. Life is 10 percent what happens to you and 90 percent how you react to it. You may not be able to banish stress from your life completely (especially if you're a natural worrier or you simply can't change the cause of your stress), but this book will teach you how to deal with stress successfully and live a far more peaceful life.

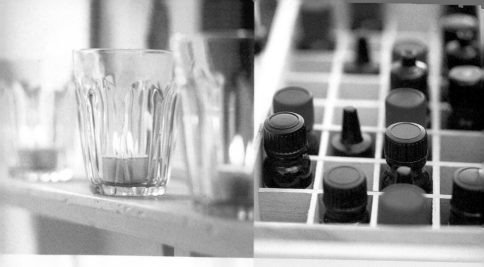

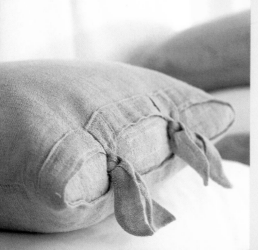

As you walk and eat and travel, be where you are. Otherwise you will miss most of your life.

Buddha

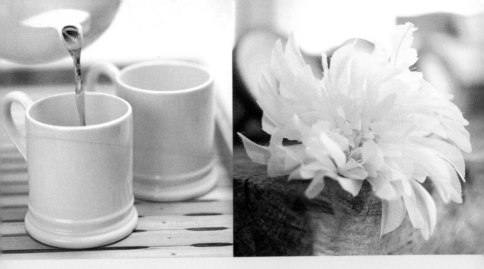

calm your body

He who is in a hurry rides on a donkey.

German proverb

exercise

Exercise not only helps you cope with current stress, it also protects you from stressful situations in the future. When your body's under stress, it needs reserves of strength to cope, and the best way to build up those reserves is by becoming fitter and healthier. Exercise also releases endorphins, pain-relieving hormones with a similar effect to heroin and morphine (now you know why they're addictive!). And, since you can't take your frustration out on your boss with physical violence (unfortunately), a brisk walk or bike ride will use up your excess energy. Not only will you be releasing tension, you'll also exhaust your body, so you're guaranteed a better night's sleep—no matter what else is going on in your life.

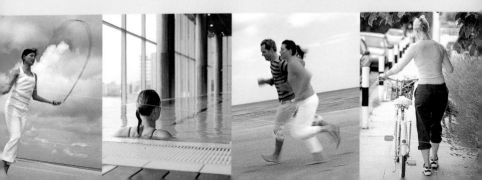

senses

Our senses are neglected during times of stress
(when the only thing you may see is your
computer screen, and the only thing you touch is
the plastic keyboard). Sensory deprivation can lead
to madness, so it's no surprise that getting back in
touch with your senses feels wonderfully relaxing.

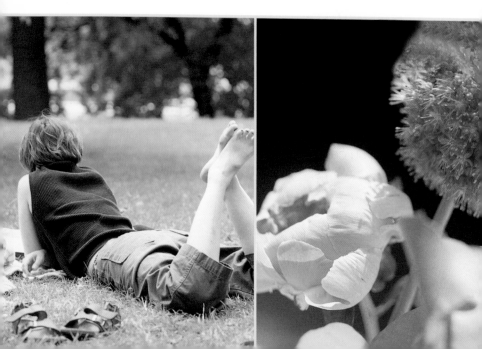

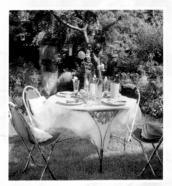

• If you spend eight hours a day in an office, make sure you go outdoors in the **DAYLIGHT** (preferably in plant-filled spaces, which are proven to relax the mind) for at least an hour every day.

• The **SOUNDS** of nature are soothing, so buy a CD recording of water, waves, or wind rustling through the trees to play after a hard day.

• Make meals a pleasure by eating at the table so you can focus on the **TASTE** of your food, rather than shoveling it down in front of the TV.

• Many of us are desperately **TOUCH**-deprived, so show friends and family you care by giving them a hug when you meet.

• Choose flowers for your home by their **SCENT** (smell them before you buy, as many flowers look pretty but are unscented).

relaxation exercise

It's easier to relax your body completely
if you first know how it feels to be tense.
For this relaxation exercise, sit in a
comfortable chair and breathe slowly
and evenly through your nose.

BEGINNING WITH YOUR RIGHT LEG, lift your leg off the floor, straighten the leg, and hold it still for 10 seconds before bending it again, and lowering it down. Repeat with the other leg.

Next, clench your buttocks as hard as you can and hold for another slow count of 10.

Clench your right fist tight and raise your arm straight out in front of you. Hold, lower it, and repeat on the other side.

Now, raise your shoulders towards your ears, tense them, and hold for 10 seconds before relaxing them down.

Scrunch up your face tight, clenching your teeth together, and squeezing your eyes shut. Hold, and then relax. With each exhale, relax your muscles a little more and enjoy the feeling of your body getting heavier.

good nutrition

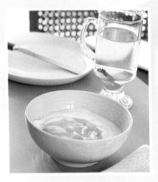

Good nutrition is essential in times of stress as your body uses up its reserves of vitamins B and C and zinc. Fill up on green vegetables, dried and fresh fruit, and whole-grain cereals, plus nuts and seeds to replace vitamin B; citrus fruits to replace vitamin C; and dairy products, red meat, and shellfish for zinc. Vitamin B also metabolizes alcohol and sugary foods, so your levels of vitamin B may be even lower if your habit is to reach for a glass of wine or a sugary snack during tough times.

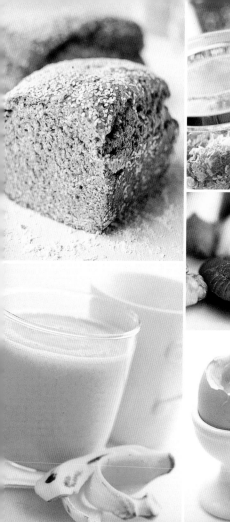
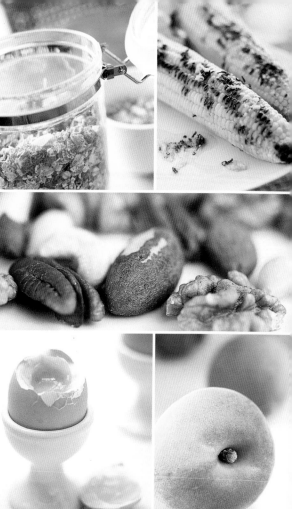

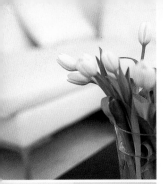

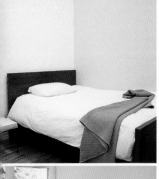

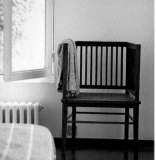

color

Color therapists believe our bodies have seven main energy centers, which are directly affected by color. Keep your surroundings calm (even when you aren't) with shades of blue and green, which are believed to help lower blood pressure and reduce your heart rate. Buy flowers for your desk or hang up a peaceful picture, and choose clothing in relaxing colors if you know the day ahead may be stressful. Most importantly, avoid red, which is the color of speed (the reason fast food restaurants are awash with the color!).

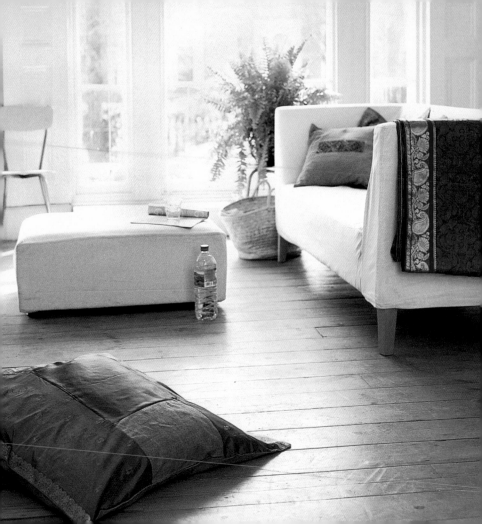

aromatherapy

As you inhale aromatherapy oils, tiny molecules are absorbed into your bloodstream, affecting your mood. Lavender is the scent most connected with safe and comforting memories, and studies show it has the power to calm and relax us in even the most stressful situations. Add five drops to your bath water or to the melted wax of a burning candle (cheaper than a vaporizer).

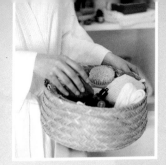

MASSAGE using essential oils equals a relaxation extravaganza! Not only does your skin draw the oils into your bloodstream, but deep breathing means you also inhale the oils, and massage movements ease tight muscles and release tension. Add five drops to two teaspoons of carrier oil (wheat germ oil, grapeseed oil, or soybean oil are best—olive oil has too strong a smell) and rub between your palms before smoothing over your skin.

meditation

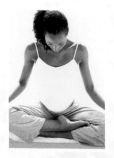

Meditation may sound new age, but it's really just a step on from deep breathing. Transcendental Meditation was founded by Maharishi Mahesh Yogi and has been found to reduce stress levels significantly. The technique is very simple. Just repeat a personal mantra in your head (any two-syllable word will do—preferably one that means nothing to you), and this word will help drive other thoughts out of your mind. When outside thoughts break into your meditation, rather than get frustrated with your scattered mind, simply acknowledge them and return to your mantra. Aim to meditate for 15–20 minutes (a perfect way to while away your commute to work), and notice how your heartbeat and breathing slow down almost immediately.

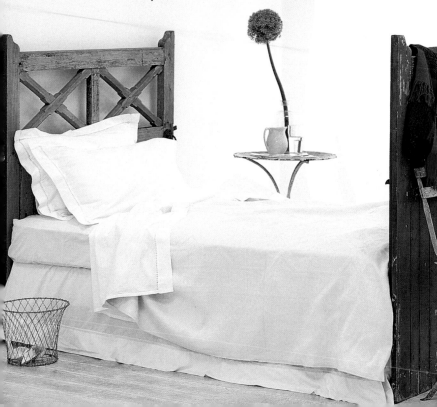

The first wealth is health.

Ralph Waldo Emerson

7 steps to starting your day in a peaceful way

1   Start the day as you mean to go on. A rushed morning routine will stress you out before you've even left the house. An extra half-hour in bed will make little difference to your day, but 30 minutes spent playing your favorite CD or eating a special breakfast can affect your mood all day.

2   What can you enjoy today? Before you get up, mentally run through your day and plan at least five pleasurable things you can fit into your busy schedule. That way, no matter how challenging your day, you can always find at least five reasons to get out of bed.

3   Still prone, stretch out as if you were trying to touch all four corners of the bed. Then bring your knees into your chest and give yourself a big hug to get rid of any stiffness in your lower back and shoulders.

4   What are the morning activities that guarantee you a good start to the day? Your clothes laid out the night before? A swim before work? Make time to do the things that set you up for a great day.

5 Just because there's no time for a bath doesn't mean you can't benefit from an aromatherapy boost. Sprinkle a few drops of bergamot oil onto your shower floor before you shower to start the day in an upbeat mood.

6 Natural chemicals in food change your mood by influencing chemicals in your brain. Protein revs you up, and carbohydrate slows you down by releasing serotonin, a mood-enhancing hormone that encourages your body to relax. Whole-wheat toast and cereal (and bananas) are all rich in serotonin-producing carbohydrates, and warm milk will also help relax muscles (the perfect excuse for an early morning latte). And pack an apple for those tense no-appetite days, as their scent has been found to ease nervous feelings.

7 Keep your keys on a hook by the front door and your handbag uncluttered. Searching for lost items equals an adrenaline rush that can easily be avoided.

When people will not
weed their own minds,
they are apt to be
overrun with nettles.
Horace Walpole

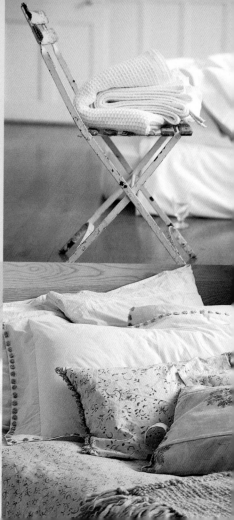

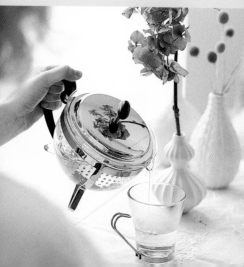

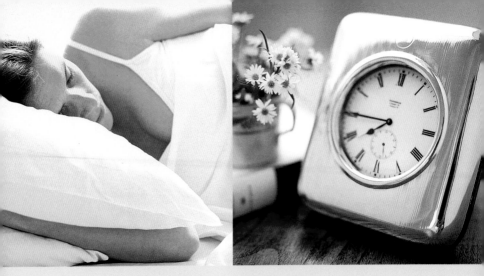

ease your mind

change how you think

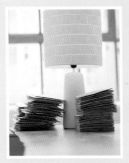

Stress is caused by feeling you don't have a choice—that there are things you *must* do and that in some way you don't want to do them. But you do have a choice, if only in your perception. Imagine a task that causes you stress. Do you really have to do it? What's the worst that can happen if you don't? Could you cope? And if there really would be serious consequences, how can you think differently about the situation to make it more bearable? Studying for an exam may be stressful, but if the qualification is going to get you a better job with more money and shorter hours, the short-term effort is probably well worth it.

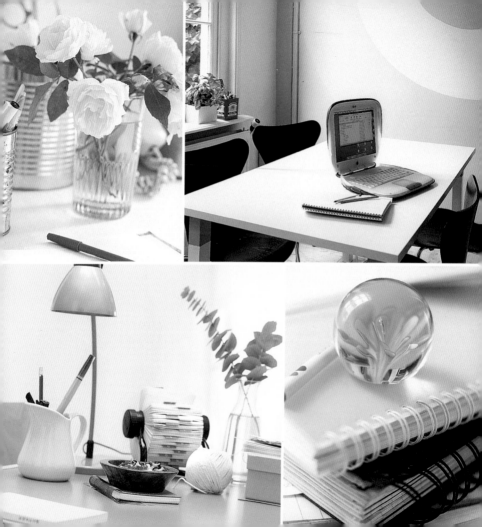

Stress is felt in your mind before it reaches your body. You can only ever hold six thoughts in your head—any more and your mind freezes like a computer with memory overload. Begin your day by deciding on your **TOP PRIORITIES**. What is most important to accomplish

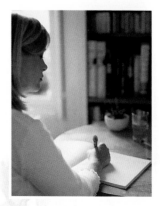

today? Write them down and only allocate your time to things that will bring you closer toward achieving these goals. You'll be amazed how much you get done with this kind of single focus.

And instead of ending your day by compiling yet another to-do list, write a **DONE LIST** of all the things you've achieved that day. Far more satisfying—and much less stressful.

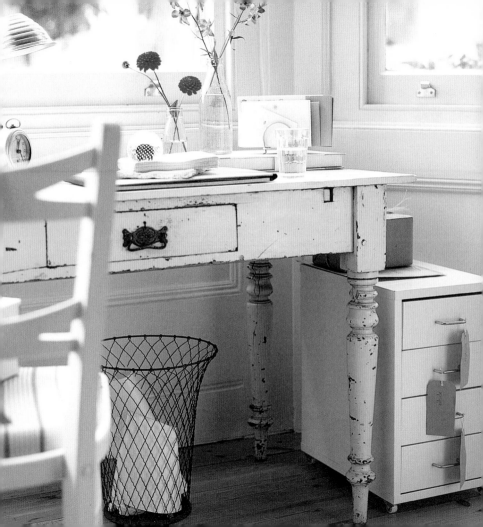

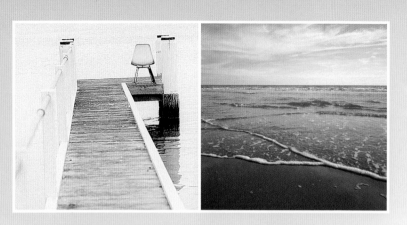

No one has ever lain on their deathbed
wishing they'd spent more time at work.
A more common regret is not appreciating
what they had. And the most likely cause?
Being too busy to notice. Remove the
sense of **URGENCY** from your life. Have you
ever asked yourself why you're rushing, only
to discover that there's no reason at all?
The next time you're stressed, notice how
you feel and make a conscious decision
to slow down. Slow your walk, slow your
speech, and take a deep breath.

Most of us take ourselves and our decisions far too **SERIOUSLY**. But rarely is anything *that* important. The next time you get stressed, ask yourself whether it really matters. Is the situation merely irritating rather than life-threatening? Will it still seem important in a month? In a week? Most situations aren't nearly as serious as we think they are and, even if this one is, one thing's guaranteed. You will only make yourself feel worse by getting upset about it.

We believe other people stress us out, when in fact we create our own feelings. So it makes sense that since we've talked ourselves into feeling this way, we can

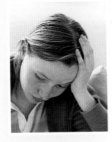

TALK OURSELVES OUT OF IT, too. If your ultimate goal is peace of mind, you first need to get over the idea that you must always have your own way—and that if you don't, you'll get upset with the person or situation that's frustrated you. Getting stressed just distracts you from finding a solution to the problem. So do yourself a favor and concentrate on ways to change the situation so it doesn't happen again. Stress has never solved a problem—only intelligence can do that.

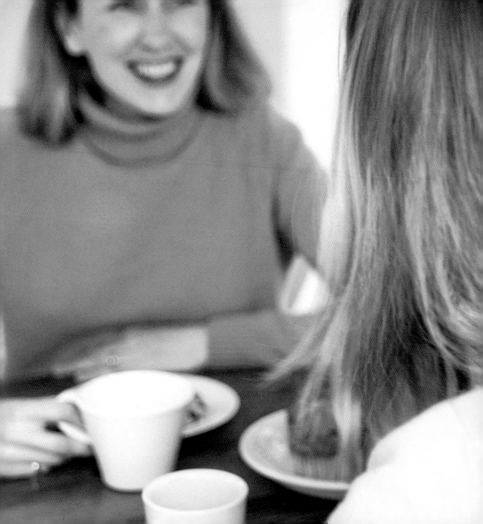

where does your time go?

You control time, not the other way around. Most of us feel a victim of shortage of time, when in reality everyone has the same 24 hours in the day and you choose how you spend yours. Are you using time wisely? How many hours this week have you spent on activities that have no meaning to you, then complained that you have no time for yourself? Aren't *you* more important?

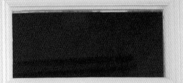

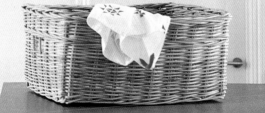

Relaxing is not the same as collapsing.
There's a big difference between free time
and **WASTED TIME**. Free time is time taken
consciously to relax and do things that feel
good. Wasted time is doing anything that
mindlessly passes the time of day. Where
are you wasting your time? Hours of TV,
chatrooms, computer games, gossiping,
crossword puzzles, complaining? This is
time which could be spent doing something
that feeds your heart.

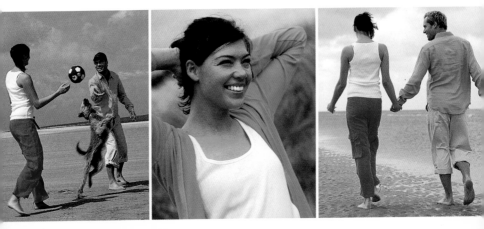

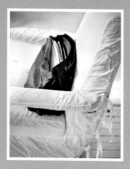

If your life is always stressful, you may be unconsciously making it so. **WHAT DRIVES YOU TO BE SO BUSY?** Do you feel guilty ("how can I relax with so much to do?"), competitive ("how can I relax when everyone else is so busy?") or ambitious ("how can I be successful if I have free time?")? Being busy doesn't earn you respect—having time for others does that. What if you were to make quality of life your number one priority? How would that change your achiever fever? Think about it: if you're not enjoying life, what's the point?

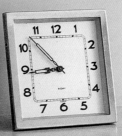

One never notices what has been done; one can only see what remains to be done.

Marie Curie

banish interruptions

Cell phones are a great way to stay busy. We think nothing of answering our phone while in the middle of a conversation, yet how rude would it be if someone just came up and started talking to your companion? Wouldn't you feel angry at being interrupted? It's better manners (and far less stressful) to switch your phone over to voicemail and fully concentrate on the person in front of you.

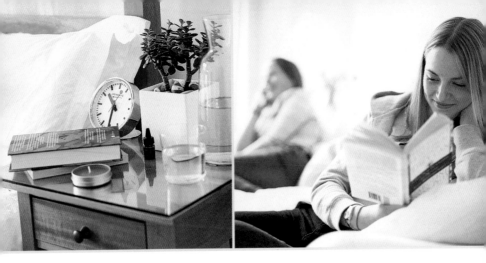

Most of us cure a stressful day by slumping in front of the TV, but the only way to completely **SILENCE INTERNAL CHATTER** is to do something that concentrates the mind, whether that's reading a book, following a recipe, or playing a musical instrument. When your mind is running exhaustive rings around you, find something to fully divert its attention.

high-octane habits

For some of us, stress is simply a way of life. But living this way is just a habit, and habits can be broken. The first step is recognizing your stress style.

Beware **ADRENALINE ADDICTION**—its effects are similar to taking speed and just as dangerous. Recognize the symptoms? Arriving late or in the nick of time, starting the next project before the last one's finished, insisting on an immediate response—and delays drive you insane, procrastinating and then rushing to deliver. Addicts often seek out professions or situations that feed their addiction, so if your life's one big drama, slow down and ask yourself if you really enjoy all this running around. And cut down your consumption of coffee and sugary snacks —they're just fueling your internal fire.

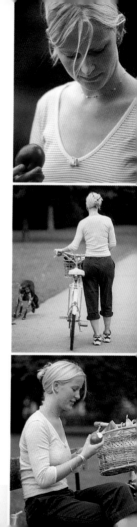

STRESS JUNKIES create more work for themselves—which then makes them even more stressed! Do you rush what's in front of you and have to repeat mistakes, rather than doing your best the first time? Do you take on everything, rather than delegating (with clear instructions) to others? Do you spend your days in crisis management, rather than responding to problems as they come up, which would save you hours? Step back and get a little perspective. There's nearly always a simpler way to do things.

Being a **PERFECTIONIST** means guaranteed stress, as you're always striving for the impossible. You know you can't really be perfect, so why not accept minor imperfections in your life? Think of someone you respect. Are they perfect? Probably not, but you still admire them. Instead, replace perfectionism with pride and commit to doing your best. Far more achievable—and enjoyable.

7 questions to ask yourself when you're stressed

1   Why am I trying to do everything myself?
What am I getting out of being a martyr?

2   What can I do to make this situation better?
How can I change the way I see it so it
becomes less stressful?

3   Where is my time best spent today? What's
the most important thing I can do right now?

4 What can I learn from this situation so I make sure I'm never put under this kind of stress again?

5 Does this really have to be done *right now*? Does the person pressuring me have something to gain from my taking instant action?

6 Is this something that will have a serious effect on my life in two weeks'/two months' time? Is it really *that* important?

7 What is my adrenaline-fueled lifestyle costing me? How quickly do I want to use up my life?

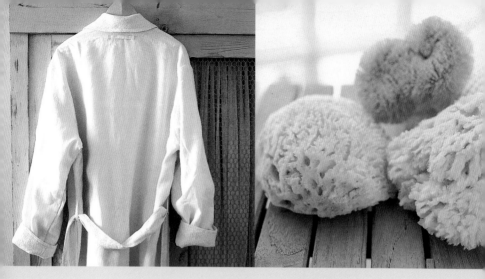

quick soothers

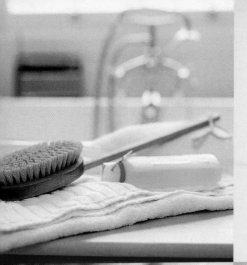

For every minute you are angry, you lose sixty seconds of happiness.

Ralph Waldo Emerson

deep breathing

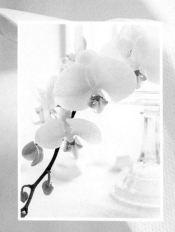

We hold stress inside our bodies by shallow breathing. It's like locking everything away in a box without giving it a chance to air. Deep breathing not only calms your senses, it revitalizes your body, too. Sit comfortably with your back straight and face relaxed. Take a great big breath in through your nose, expanding your stomach as you inhale. Imagine your body filling up with air from all directions as if you were a big balloon. Pause for a second and then slowly breathe out through your nose until your lungs feel completely empty. Repeat 5–10 times until you feel your nerves settle and still.

If your mind's racing, calm it down by **CONCENTRATING ON YOUR BREATH**: how long you can breathe in and out, and how good it feels. Don't worry if your thoughts wander. Just gently bring them back to your breath and your mind will gradually slow down to match its rhythm.

limber up

A big stretch will loosen up tense muscles, and lengthening your spine not only feels fantastic, it also enables you to breathe more deeply. Lie on your back with your arms stretched out over your head. Interlock your fingers, point your toes, take a big inhalation and stretch your arms and legs away from you. Hold for a few seconds, relax, and repeat five times.

SHIATSU MASSAGE works on the meridians in your body to influence the energy flowing through you. Along each meridian are points where the flow can be most easily influenced. To find your stress-relief point, slide your thumb between the bones leading to your middle and ring fingers until you've reached the center of your palm. Breathe in and press into this point with your thumb as you slowly breathe out (if you've hit the right spot, you'll feel a dull ache). For best results, press and hold six times on each hand.

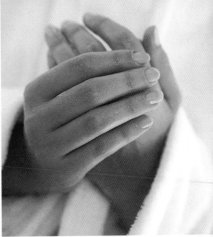

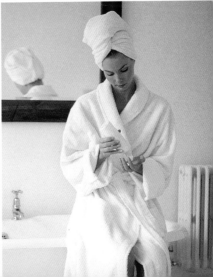

sound and vision

Noise pollution may be part of the
problem, but the right sounds can
reduce stress by releasing a hormone
that helps to control the production
of adrenaline. Music can also trigger
the release of feel-good endorphins,
so put together a CD or cassette of
your favorite soothing sounds and
press "Play" after a busy day.

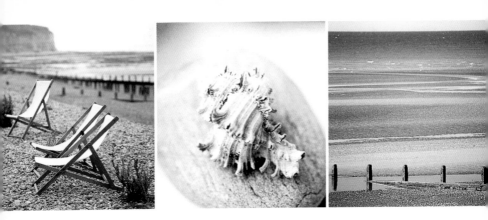

Take yourself away from the madness with a few minutes of **VISUALIZATION**. Close your eyes and imagine you're back on vacation—lying on a deserted beach or watching the sun go down. It may sound simple, but research has shown people can control stress and even fight illness with the power of their imagination. And it sure beats staring at your fellow passengers on the commute home.

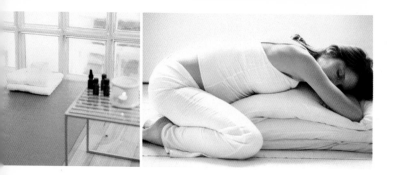

yoga

As any yoga fan will tell you, child's pose is just about the most relaxing position you can put yourself in. The pose feels so good because it calms and tones your nervous system while gently stretching your neck, shoulders, and spine. Kneel on the floor with your arms by your sides and bend forward until your forehead is gently resting on the floor in front of you and your hands are resting by your feet. Inhale and exhale as you feel your breath slow and your body completely relax. Bliss.

Not being able to breathe through one nostril for over two hours is believed to be a sign of potential illness. **ALTERNATIVE NOSE BREATHING** not only balances your breath, it calms your body, too. Place your thumb over your right nostril to close it and slowly inhale into your left nostril. Release the right nostril, use your ring finger to block the left nostril, and exhale through the right nostril. Now, stay as you are and inhale slowly into your right nostril, place your thumb back on your right nostril to block it and exhale through your left nostril. Repeat five times.

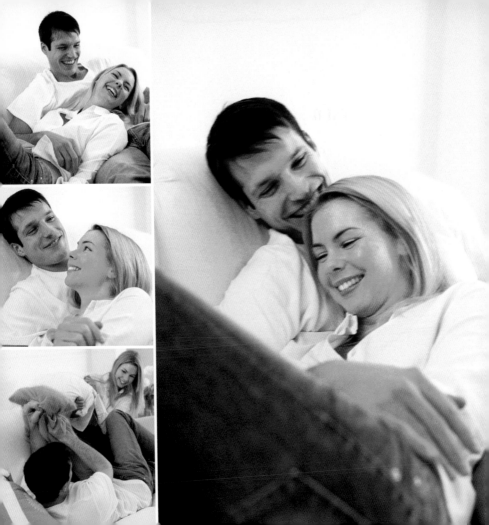

the best medicine

The next time you feel stressed, simply relax your shoulders, take a deep breath, and smile. Research shows that smiling can lower the levels of steroid chemicals in the blood associated with both physical and psychological stress.

Or go one better and **LAUGH**. Laughter releases endorphins (the ones you usually have to exercise to get) into your brain, which reduces levels of the stress hormone cortisol, relaxes tense muscles, and boosts your immune system. The average adult laughs only 17 times a day (compared to 300 times as a child), so do what it takes to lighten up. Phone a funny friend, store jokes on your computer for instant amusement, or laugh at yourself for taking life so seriously...

7 steps to fast stress relief

1 To relax tension in your neck while sitting at your desk, interlock your fingers behind your head with your elbows pointing outwards. Inhale, and as you exhale, drop your chin to your chest, bringing your elbows together in front of your face. Keep your shoulders relaxed and feel the weight of your arms gently stretching the back of your neck.

2 Feel in desperate need of a massage? You can easily do the job yourself. Rest your right elbow in your left hand and then, using your hand as support, push your right hand over your shoulder. Now you're perfectly placed to massage into the side of your spine and your shoulder blade. Finish by grasping the muscles in your shoulders and then repeat on the other side.

3 Your lower jaw is the first joint to stiffen in times of stress. Release the tension by moving your jaw from side to side, then use the first two fingers of each hand to massage the joint where the upper and lower jaws meet. Even easier—bite into an apple for an instant lower-face relaxer.

4   Tense, stressed-out headache? Gently press your first two fingers just under the bone at the base of your skull, either side of your spine. Lean back onto your fingers and then work in gentle circular movements down either side of your neck, spending a little longer on tender areas.

5   Singing and humming relieve stress as they cause relaxing vibrations in your throat. Hum to yourself when you start to feel stressed, and at the end of a busy day, turn up the car radio and sing all the way home.

6   Reflexology works on the reflex points in your feet, and massaging your adrenal gland reflexes equals instant stress relief. Situated on the soles of your feet slightly inside the middle of each arch, use your thumb held bent at a 45-degree angle and massage firmly into each reflex point for two minutes maximum.

7   You don't need to be in a calming environment to meditate effectively. Zone out by watching something repetitive like clothes in a washing machine or traffic from a bus window. Soften your focus and detach your thoughts—you may be amazed where they go when you let them wander.

resources

aromatherapy

**Atlantic Institute of
Aromatherapy**
16018 Saddlestring Drive
Tampa, FL 33612
t. 813 265 2222
www.atlanticinstitute.com

Institute of Aromatherapy
3108 Route 10 West
Denville, NJ 07834
t. 973 989 1999
www.instituteof
   aromatherapy.com

**Pacific Institute of
Aromatherapy**
P.O. Box 6723
San Rafael, CA 94903
t. 415 479 9121

stores

Aveda
t. 866 823 1425 for stores
www.aveda.com

Bath & Body Works
t. 800 395 1001 for stores
www.bathandbodyworks.com

Barneys New York
660 Madison Avenue
New York NY 10021
t. 212 826 8900
www.barneys.com

Bed Bath and Beyond
620 Sixth Avenue
New York NY 10011
t. 800 462 3966 for stores
www.bedbathandbeyond.com

Crabtree and Evelyn
t. 800 272 2873 for stores
www.crabtree-evelyn.com

Crate & Barrel
650 Madison Avenue
New York NY 10022
t. 800 967 6696 for stores
www.crateandbarrel.com

Origins
www.origins.com for stockists
and stores

Sephora
2103 Broadway
New York NY 10023
t. 212 362 1500
www.sephora.com for stores

credits

Key: ph=photographer, a=above, b=below, r=right, l=left, c=center

Endpapers ph Polly Wreford; 1 ph David Montgomery; 2 ph Polly Wreford; 3 ph Polly Wreford / Kimberley Watson's house in London; 4–5 ph Polly Wreford; 6 ph Debi Treloar / Robert Elms and Christina Wilson's family home in London (christinawilson@btopenworld.com); 7 ph Polly Wreford; 8al ph Polly Wreford; 8ar & b ph David Montgomery; 9 ph Debi Treloar; 10–11 ph Chris Everard; 11r ph Debi Treloar; 12l ph Debi Treloar; 12r ph David Brittain; 13 background ph Chris Tubbs; 13 inset ph David Brittain; 14–15 ph Polly Wreford; 16 background ph Ian Wallace; 16 inset ph David Montgomery; 17al ph Philip Webb; 17ac ph David Montgomery; 17ar ph Ian Wallace; 17c & bl ph Francesca Yorke; 17bc & br ph Debi Treloar; 18al ph Alan Williams / Jennifer & Geoffrey Symonds' apartment in New York designed by Jennifer Post Design (www.jenniferpostdesign.com); 18cl ph Polly Wreford / home of 27.12 Design Ltd, Chelsea, NYC (www.2712design.com); 18bl ph Jan Baldwin / interior designer Didier Gomez's apartment in Paris (orygomez@free.fr); 18r ph Jan Baldwin; 19 ph Polly Wreford / Kimberley Watson's house in London; 20–21 inset ph Dan Duchars; 21r ph Polly Wreford; 22 ph Debi Treloar; 23 ph Tom Leighton; 24 ph William Lingwood; 25 ph Ian Wallace; 26a ph Tom Leighton; 26bl ph Dan Duchars; 26br ph Debi Treloar / Susan Cropper's family home in London (www.63hlg.com); 27l ph Debi Treloar; 27r ph Dan Duchars; 28 ph Andrew Wood; 29al ph Polly Wreford; 29ar ph Jan Baldwin / Claire Haithwaite and Dean Maryon's home in Amsterdam; 29bl ph Dan Duchars; 29br ph Polly Wreford; 30 inset ph Dan Duchars; 30 background–31 ph Polly Wreford; 32l inset ph Jan Baldwin; 32r inset & background–33 ph Chris Tubbs; 34–35 ph Dan Duchars; 36 ph Debi Treloar; 37 ph Chris Everard; 38 background ph Catherine Gratwicke; 38 inset ph Andrew Wood / Gabriele Sanders' apartment in New York; 39 ph Polly Wreford; 40 ph Jan Baldwin / the Meiré family home, designed by Marc Meiré; 41l ph David Montgomery; 41r ph Dan Duchars; 42 ph Alan Williams; 43l ph Alan Williams / Jennifer & Geoffrey Symonds' apartment in New York designed by Jennifer Post Design (www.jenniferpostdesign.com); 43r ph Debi Treloar; 44–46 ph Polly Wreford; 47 ph Dan Duchars; 48l ph Polly Wreford; 48r ph David Montgomery; 49a ph Chris Everard; 49b ph Dan Duchars; 50 background ph Tom Leighton; 50 inset–52 ph Polly Wreford; 53l ph Andrew Wood; 53ar ph David Montgomery; 53br ph Polly Wreford; 54 ph Debi Treloar / Robert Elms and Christina Wilson's family home in London (christinawilson@btopenworld.com); 55l ph Tom Leighton; 55c ph Jan Baldwin; 55r ph Debi Treloar; 56 background ph Polly Wreford; 56l inset ph David Montgomery; 56r inset ph Debi Treloar; 57 ph Dan Duchars; 58 ph Polly Wreford; 60–61 ph Debi Treloar; 62 ph Polly Wreford; 63 ph David Brittain; 64 ph Debi Treloar.

acknowledgments

The author would like to thank
the following: Alison Starling of
Ryland Peters & Small for asking
me to write this book; Coach U
for teaching me not to accept
stress as part of my everyday
life; and all my wonderful
family and friends.

Visit Liz Wilde's website at
www.wildelifecoaching.com for
information about her one-to-one
coaching and online programs.
Her book, *Unlock Your Potential*,
is also published by
Ryland Peters & Small.

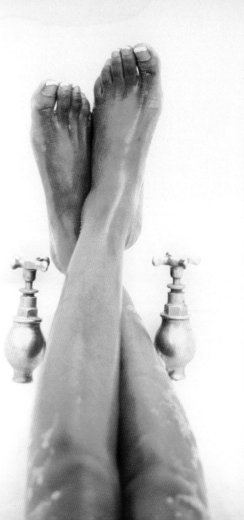

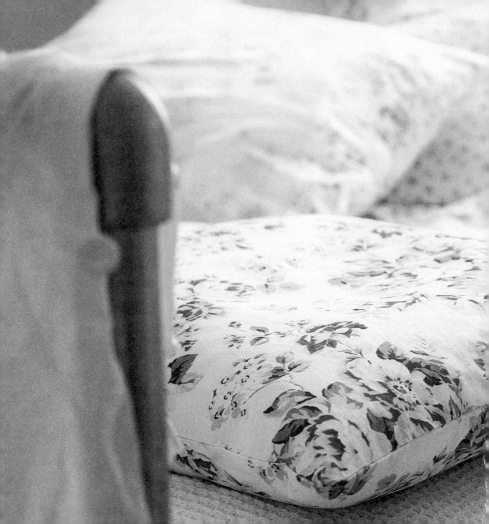